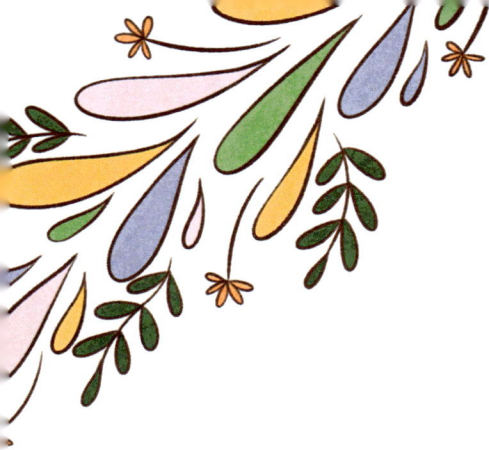

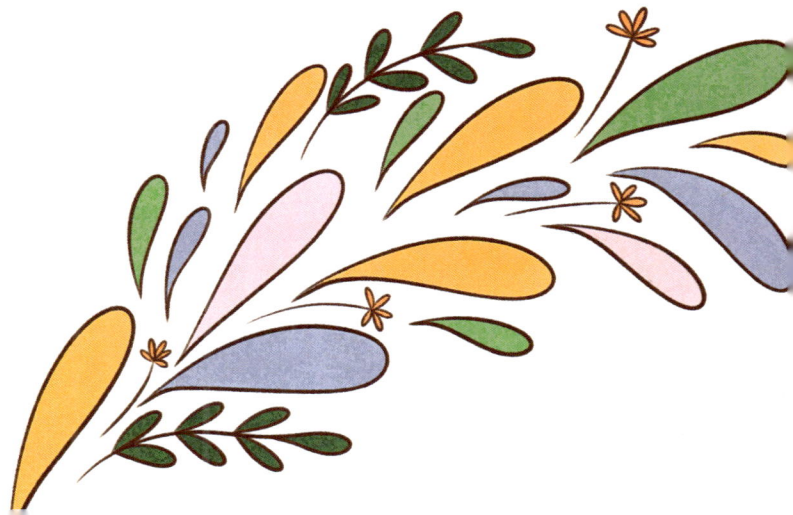

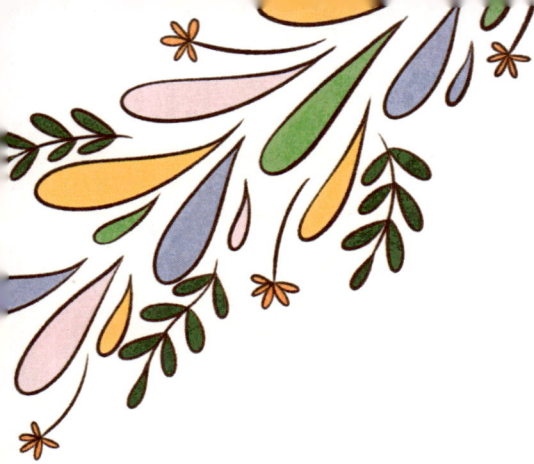

Brenda L. Hwang, M.A., CCC-SLP, CLC
Speech Garden, LLC co-founder
Collierville, Tennessee
www.speechgardentherapy.com

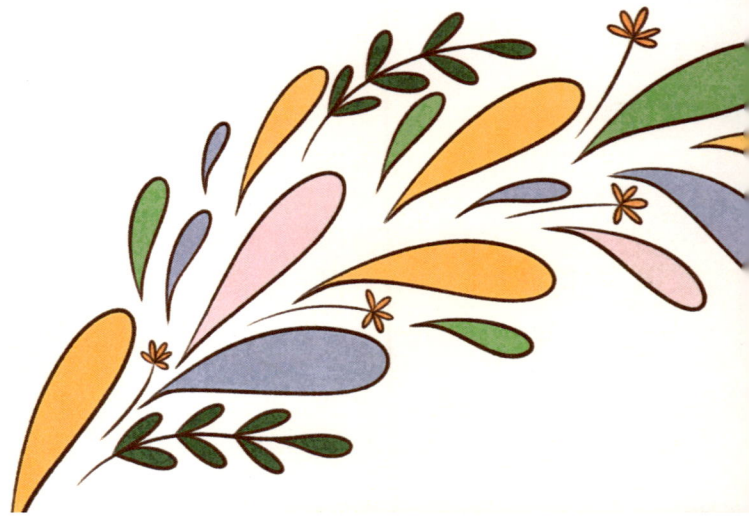

Mama,
watch me grow

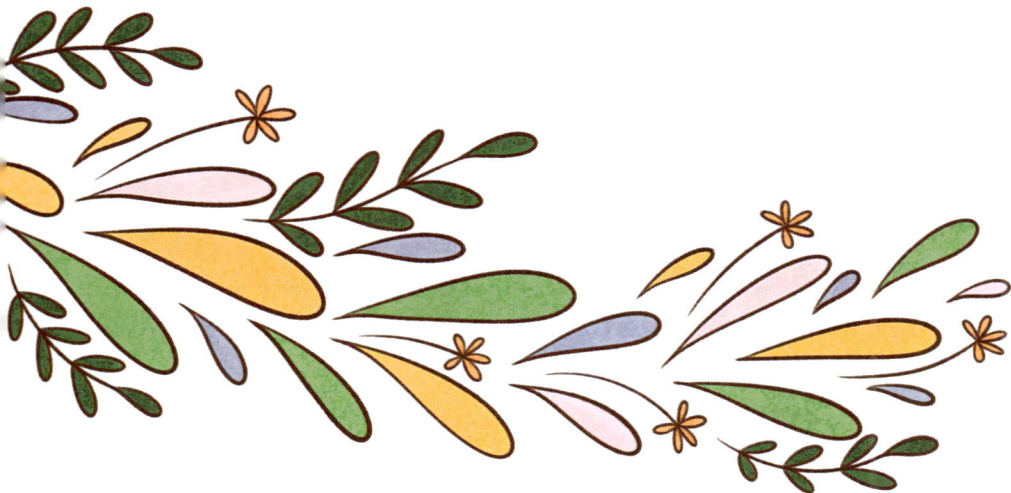

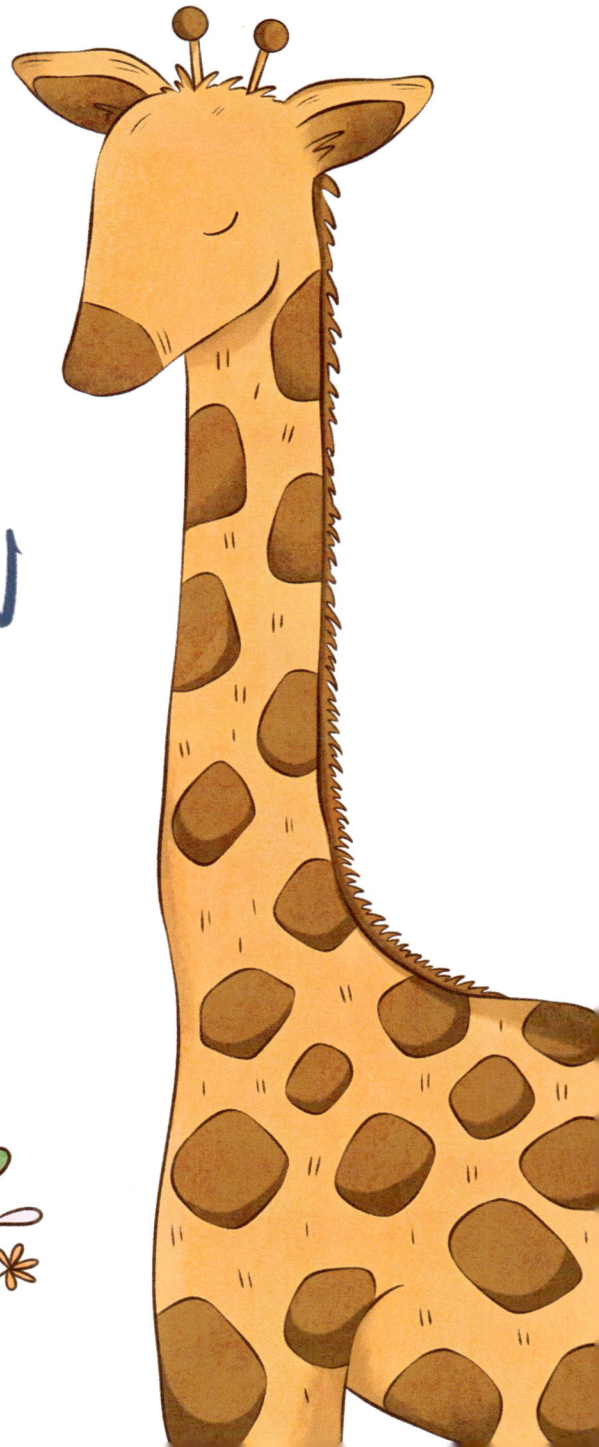

4-5 Weeks

9 Weeks

18 Weeks

24 Weeks

25-26 Weeks

27 Weeks

0-3 months

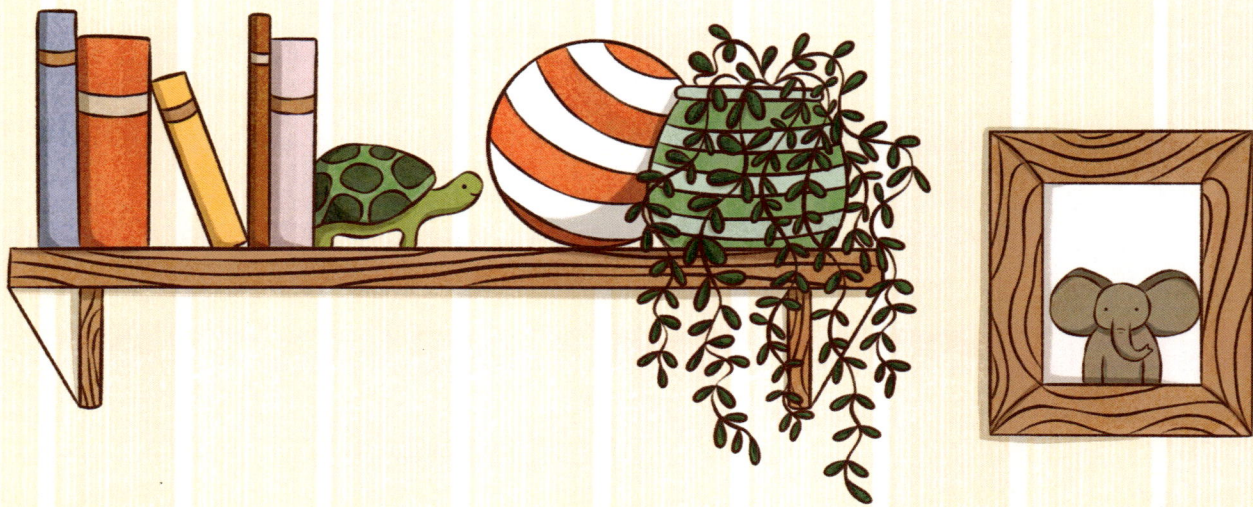

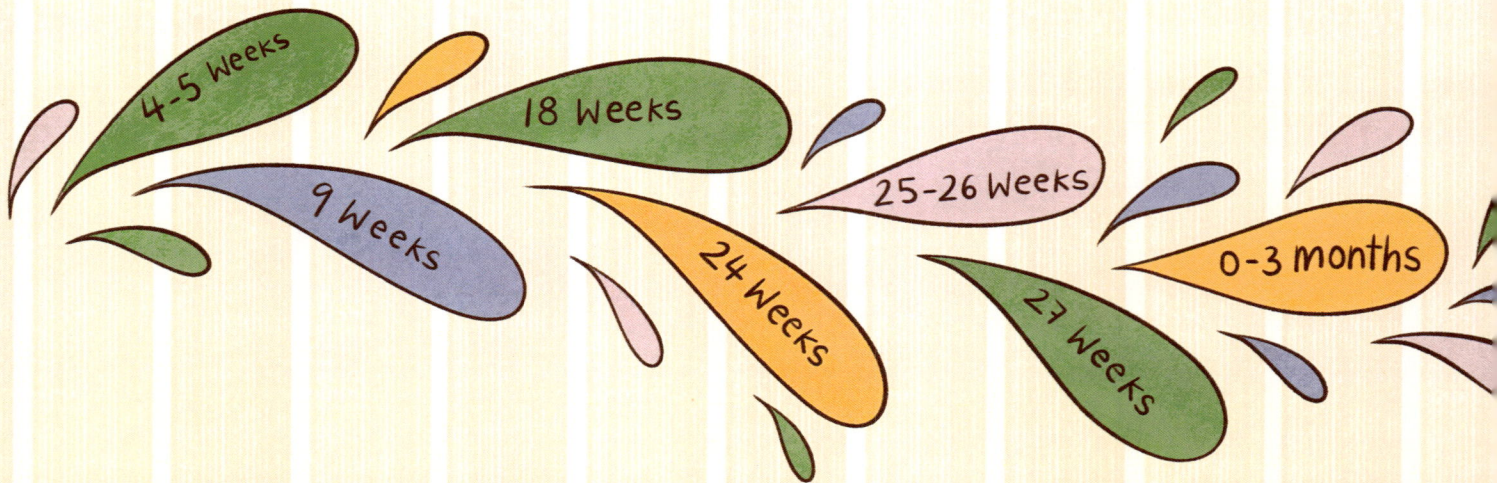

For my babies, Liam & Jane.
Mama loves to watch you both grow.

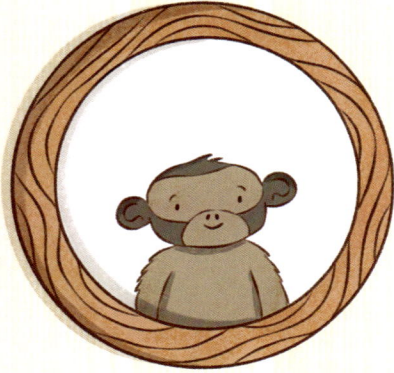
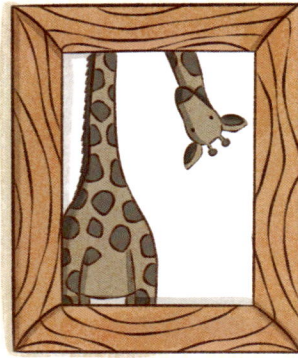

6-9 months

12-15 months

18-24 months

24-36 months

3-6 months

9-12 months

15-18 months

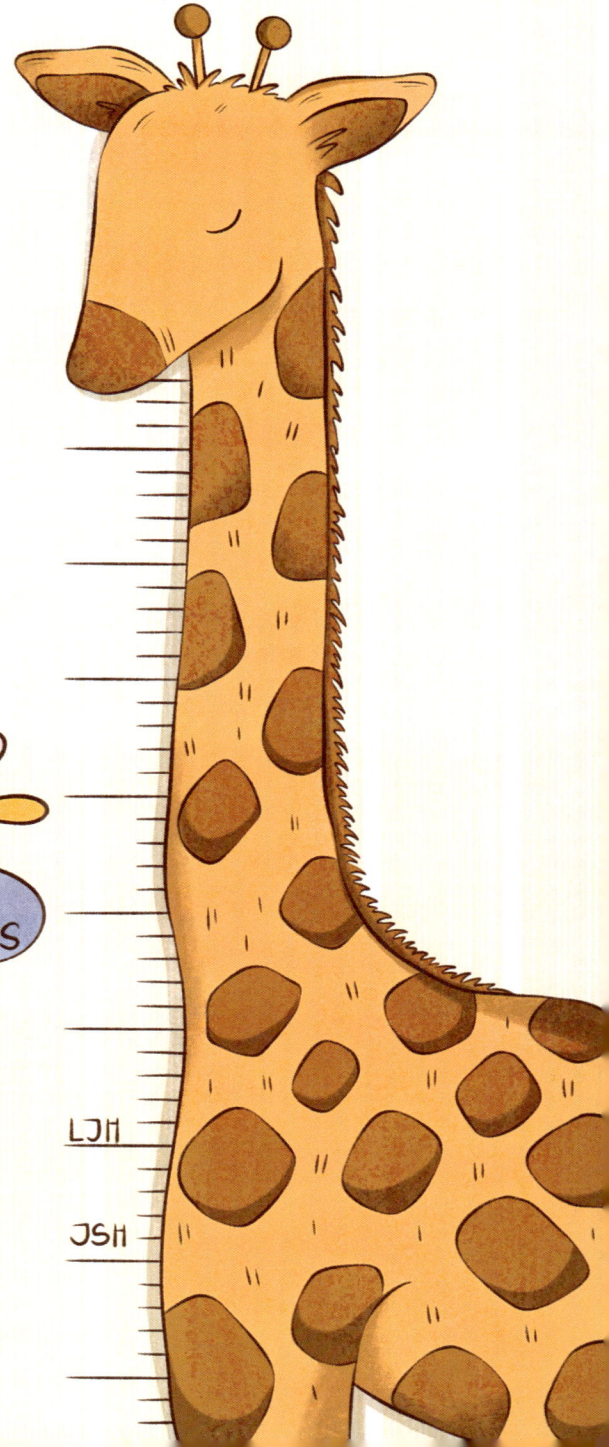

LJH

JSH

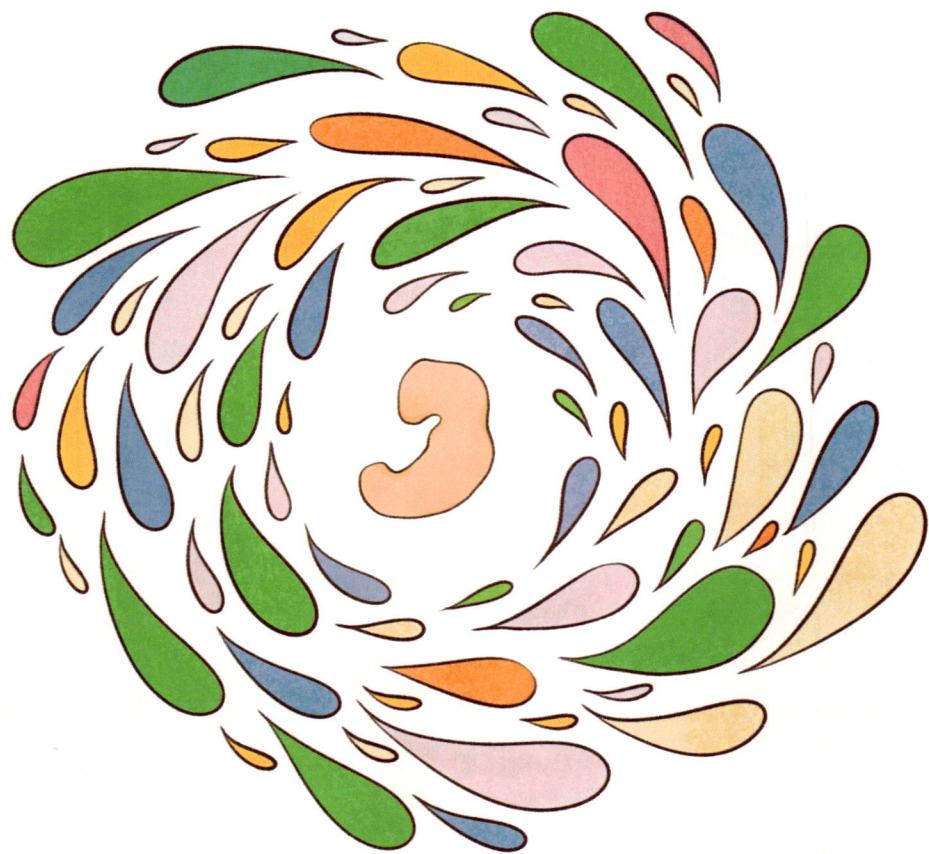

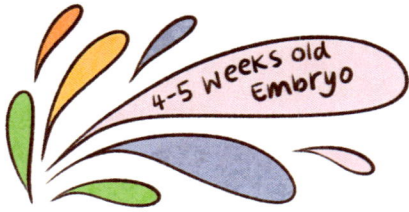

4-5 weeks old Embryo

Mama, I'm coming, though at my own pace.
This journey together, we two will embrace.
No matter if I'm fast or slow.
Come along, Mama. Watch me grow!

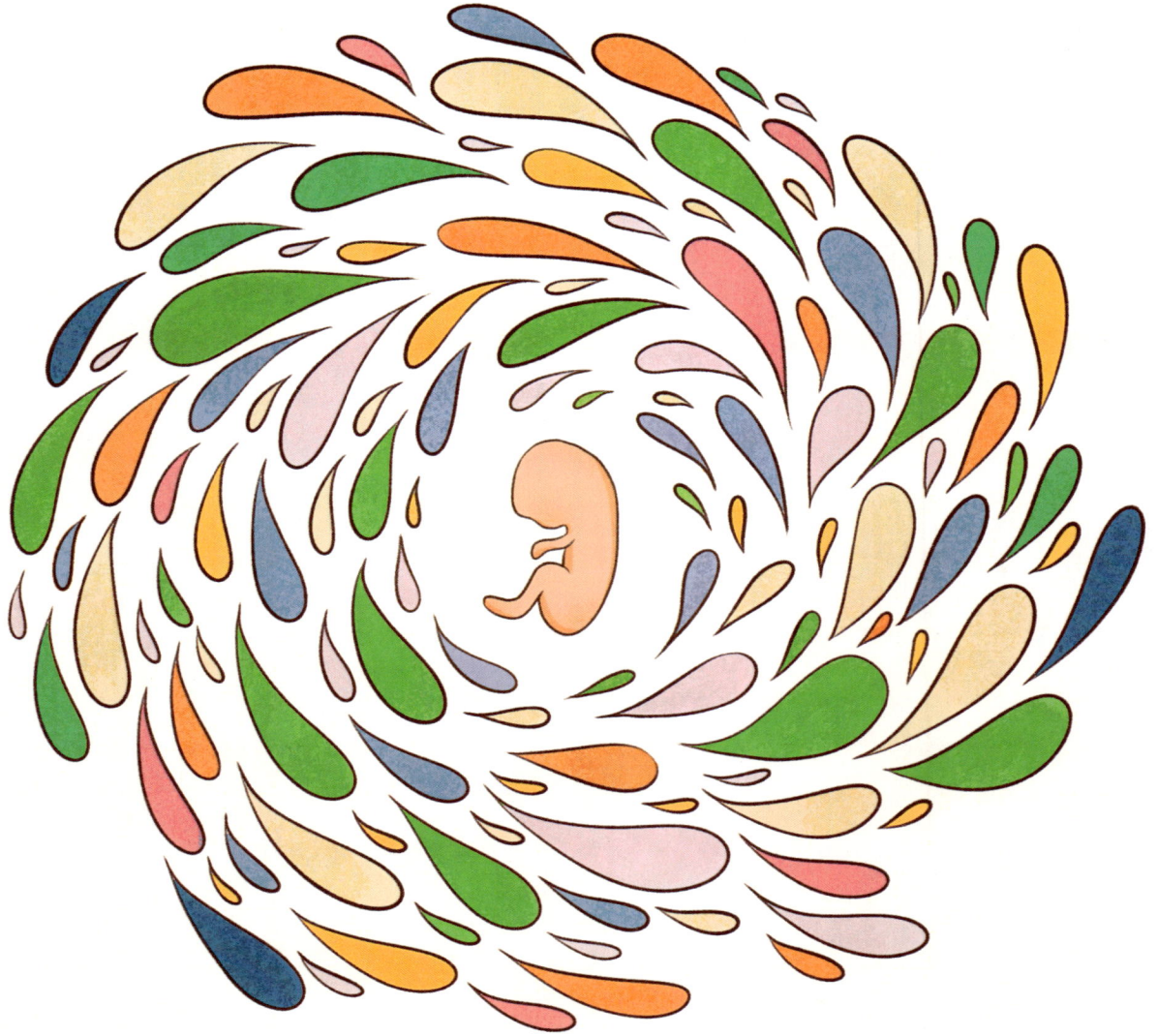

9 weeks old Embryo

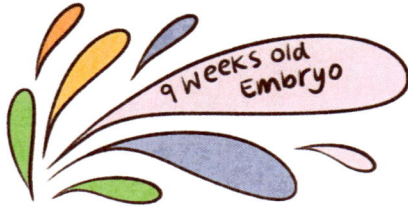

Mama, look closely, and you'll start to see,
right where my two little ears will soon be.
A cute little button, but growing a bit.
Your own mini-me, and together we fit.

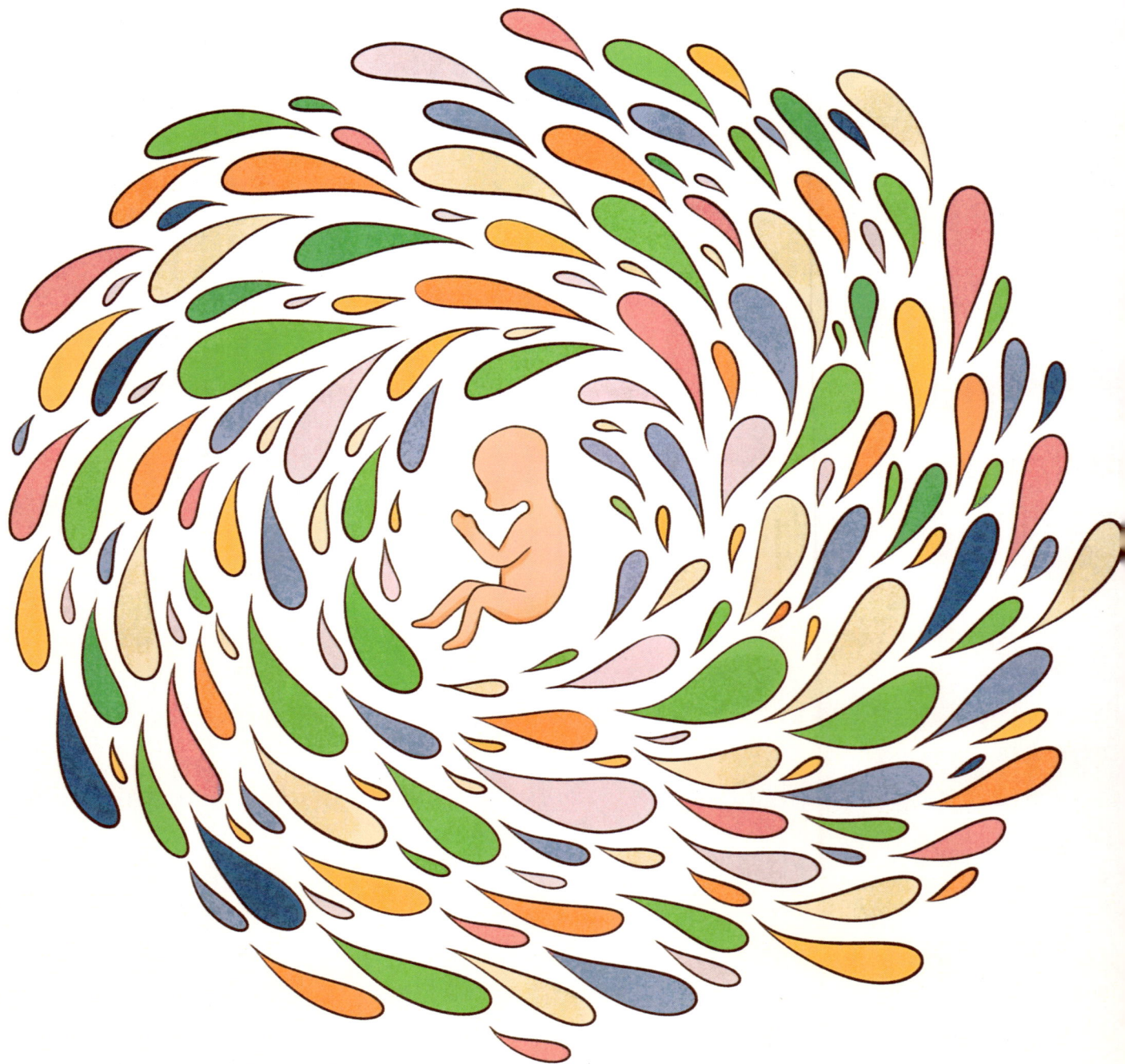

18 Weeks old
Fetus

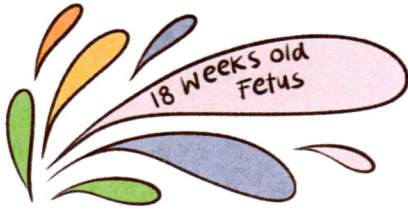

I can hear! I can hear!
What a strange little treat.
From morning till night,
I can hear your heart beat!

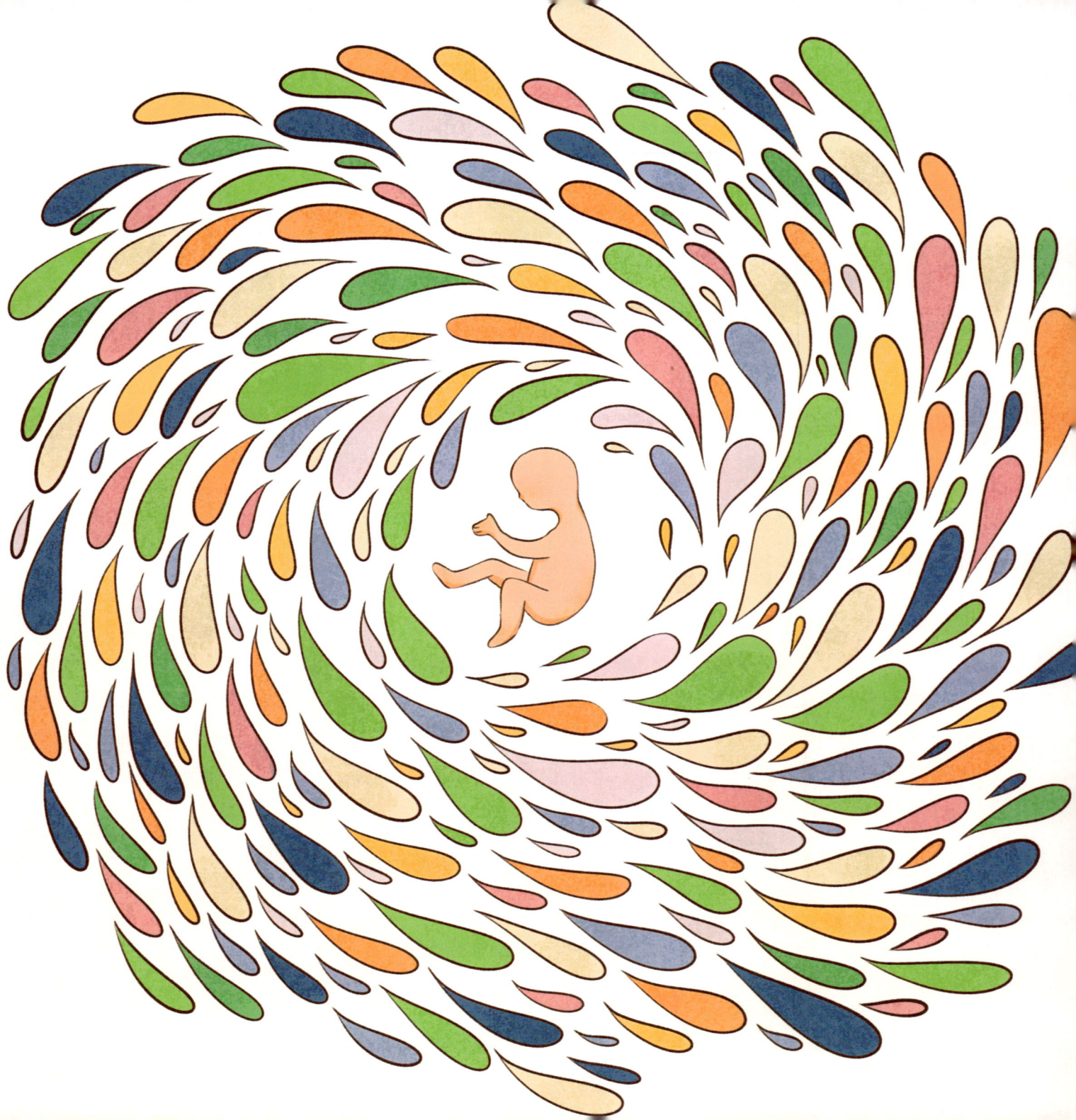

24 Weeks old
Fetus

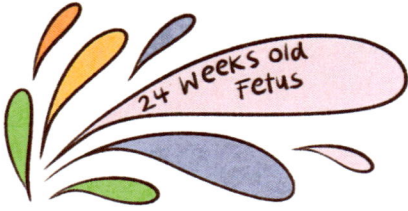

I hear muffled noises.
You're talking to me!
The sound of your voice
fills my heart up with glee.

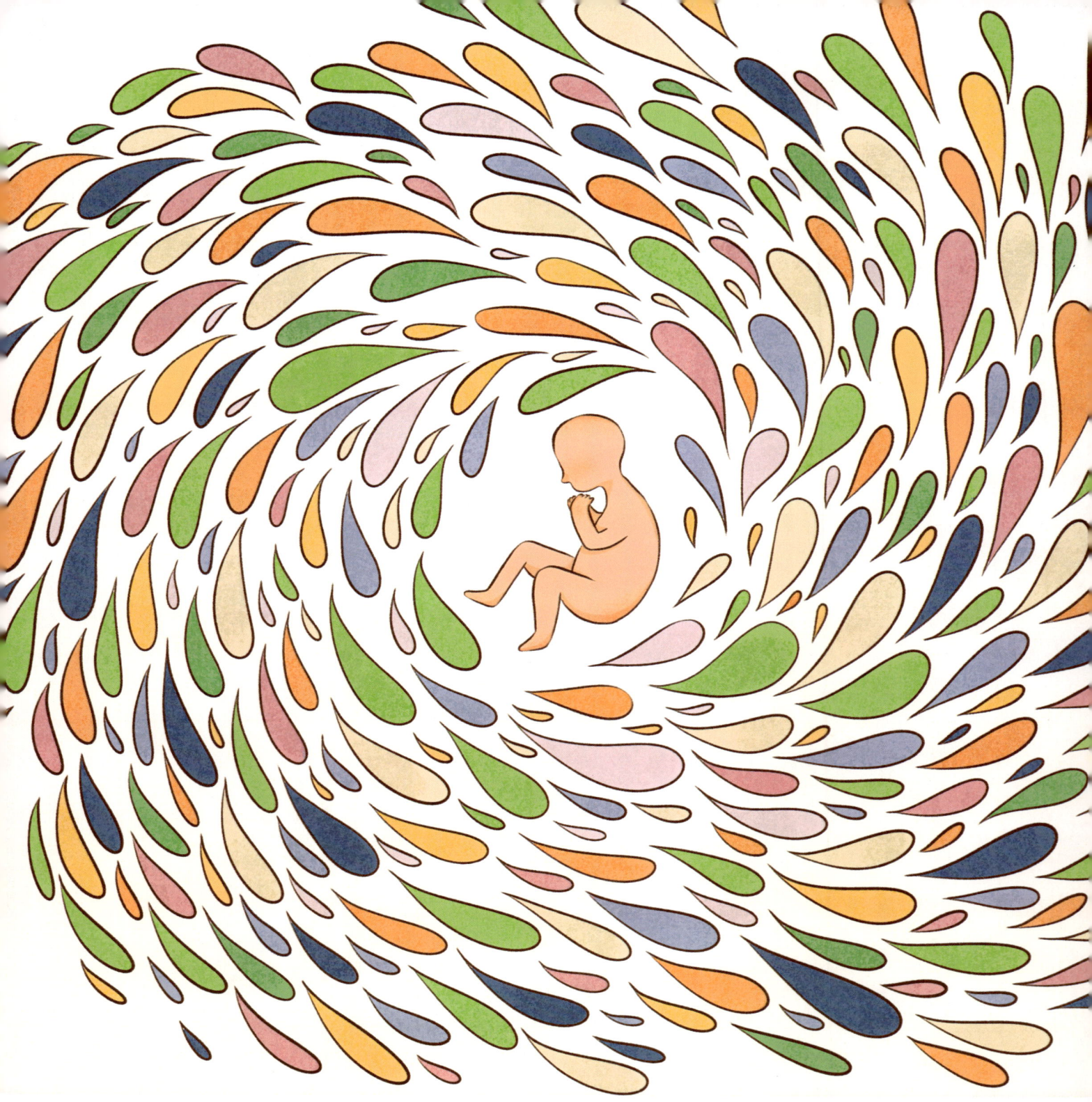

25-26 weeks old
Fetus

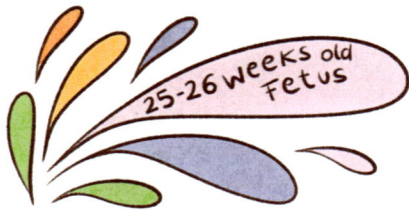

My hearing's developing more every day.
Sing to me! Talk to me!
I will hear what you say.

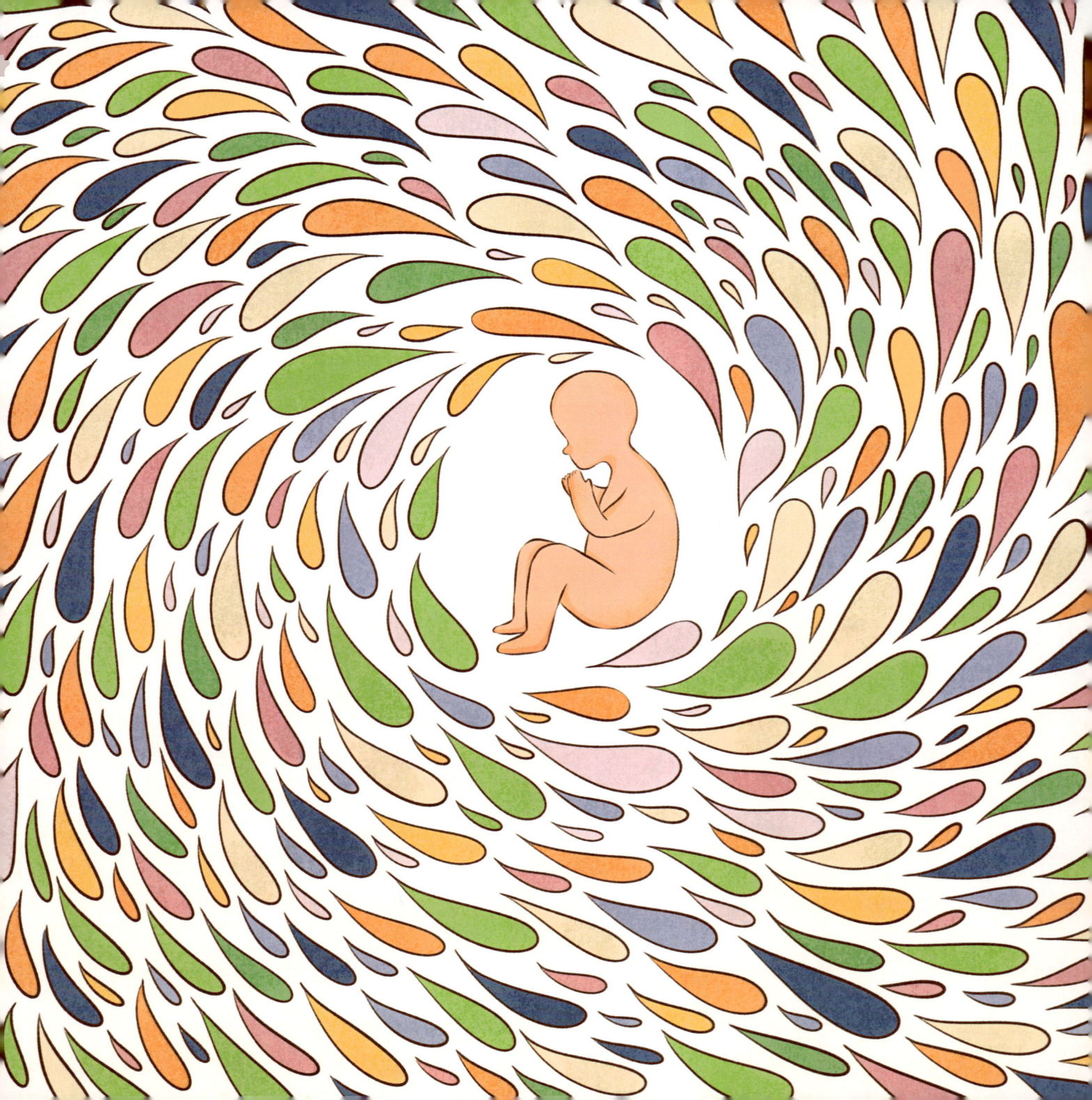

27 weeks old
Fetus

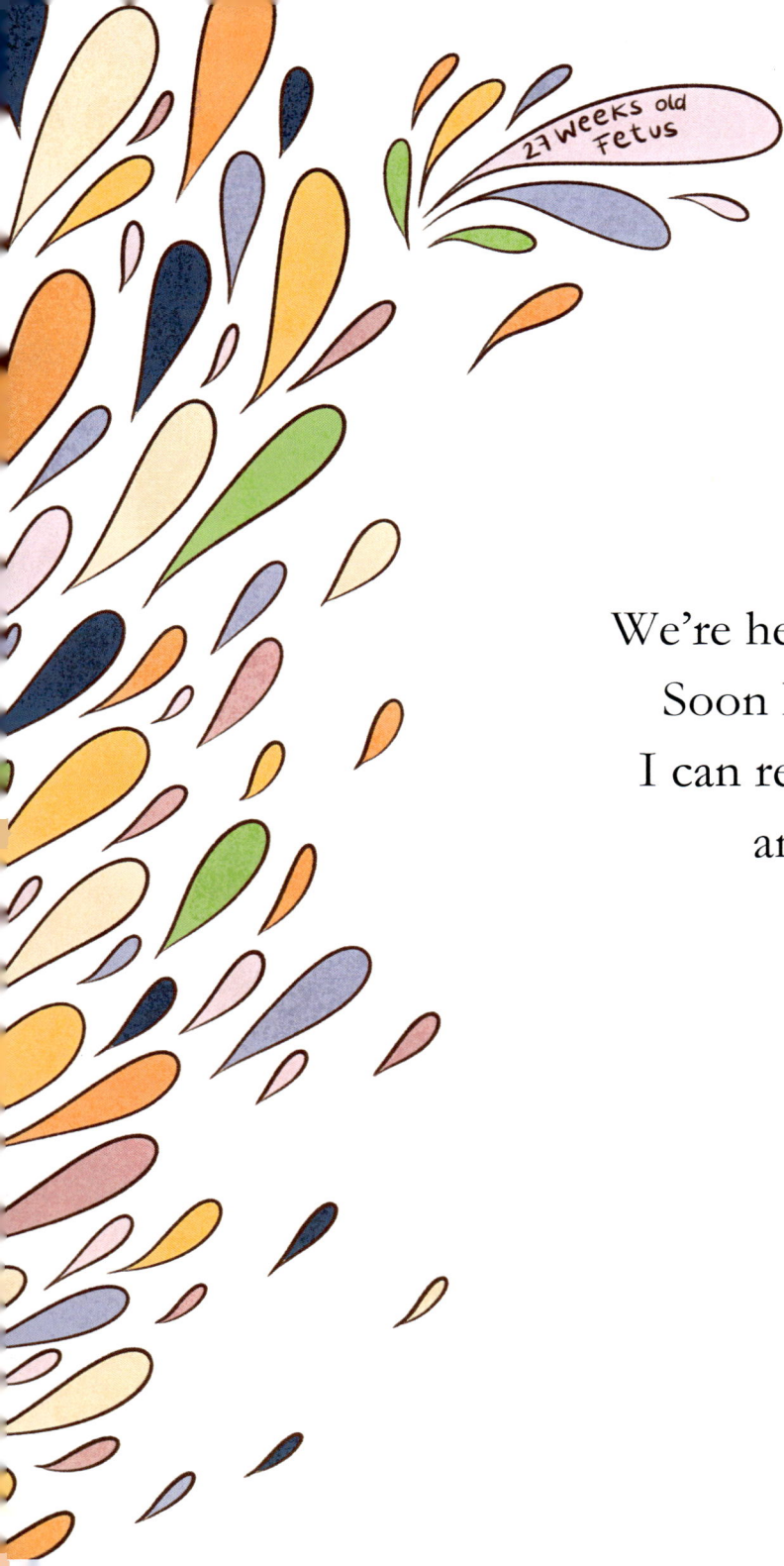

We're here in the final stretch.
Soon I'll get to meet you.
I can recognize your voice,
and daddy's too!

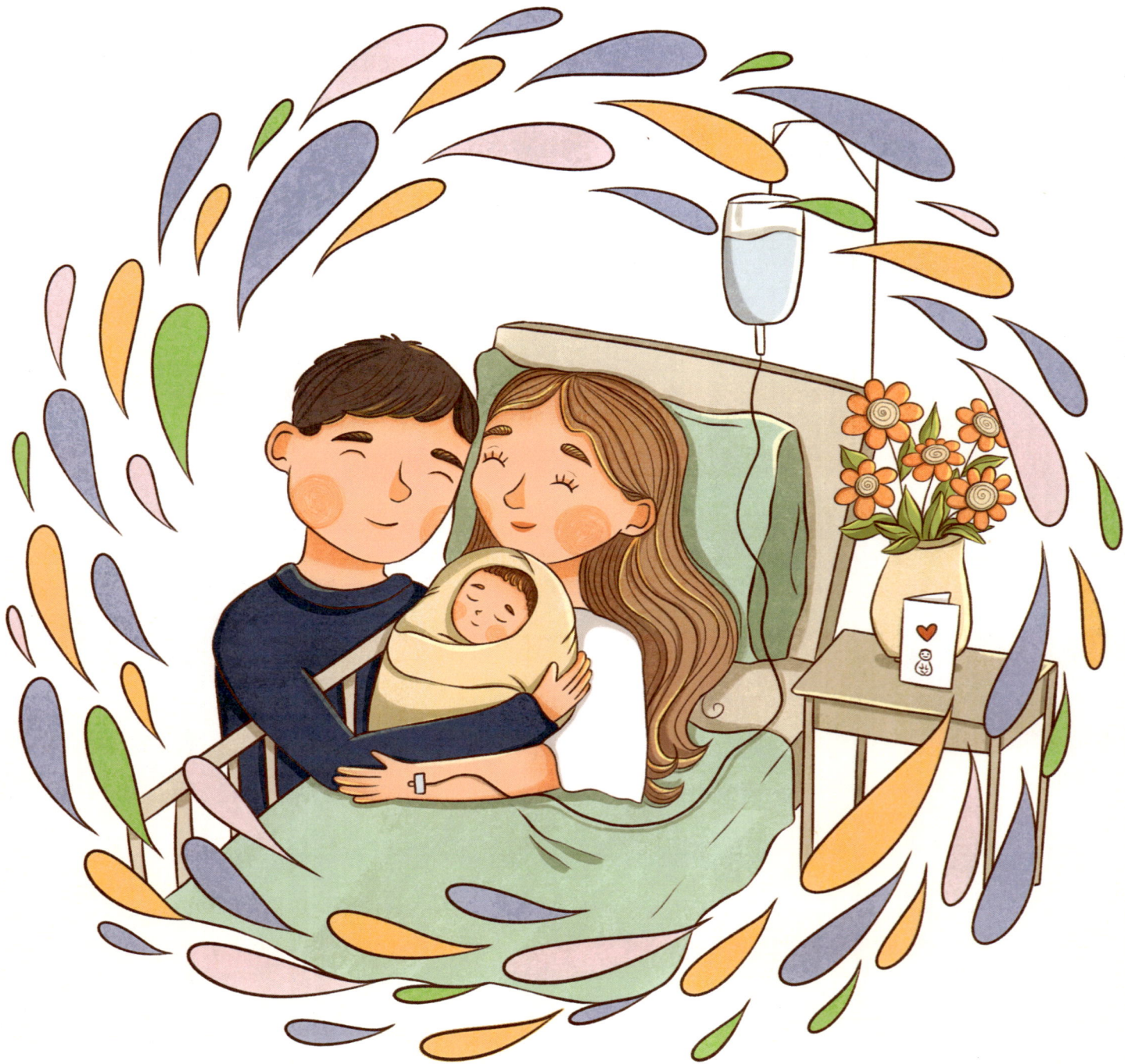

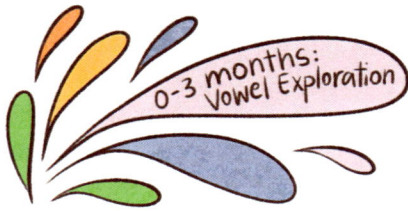

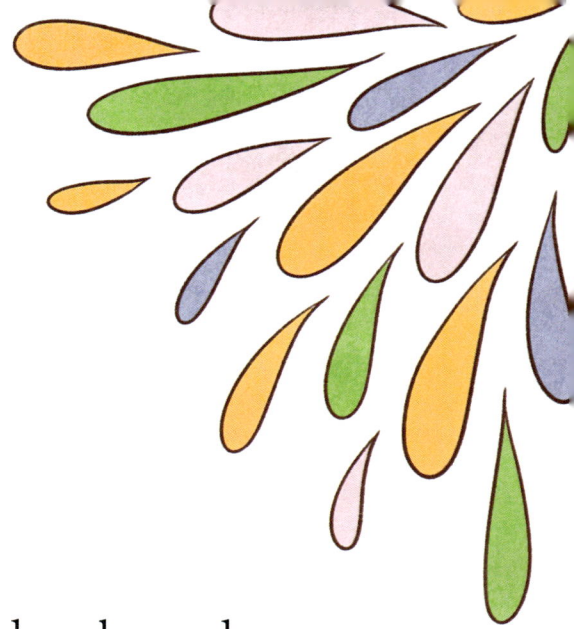

Hello, world. I'm here, and my wonder abounds.

I'm busy exploring a whole world of sounds.

I coo and I smile at life's little joys,

But startle each time that I hear a loud noise.

Contact baby's pediatrician and reach out to a speech-language pathologist at **3 months** if baby is not: responding to sounds; tracking moving objects with eye gaze.

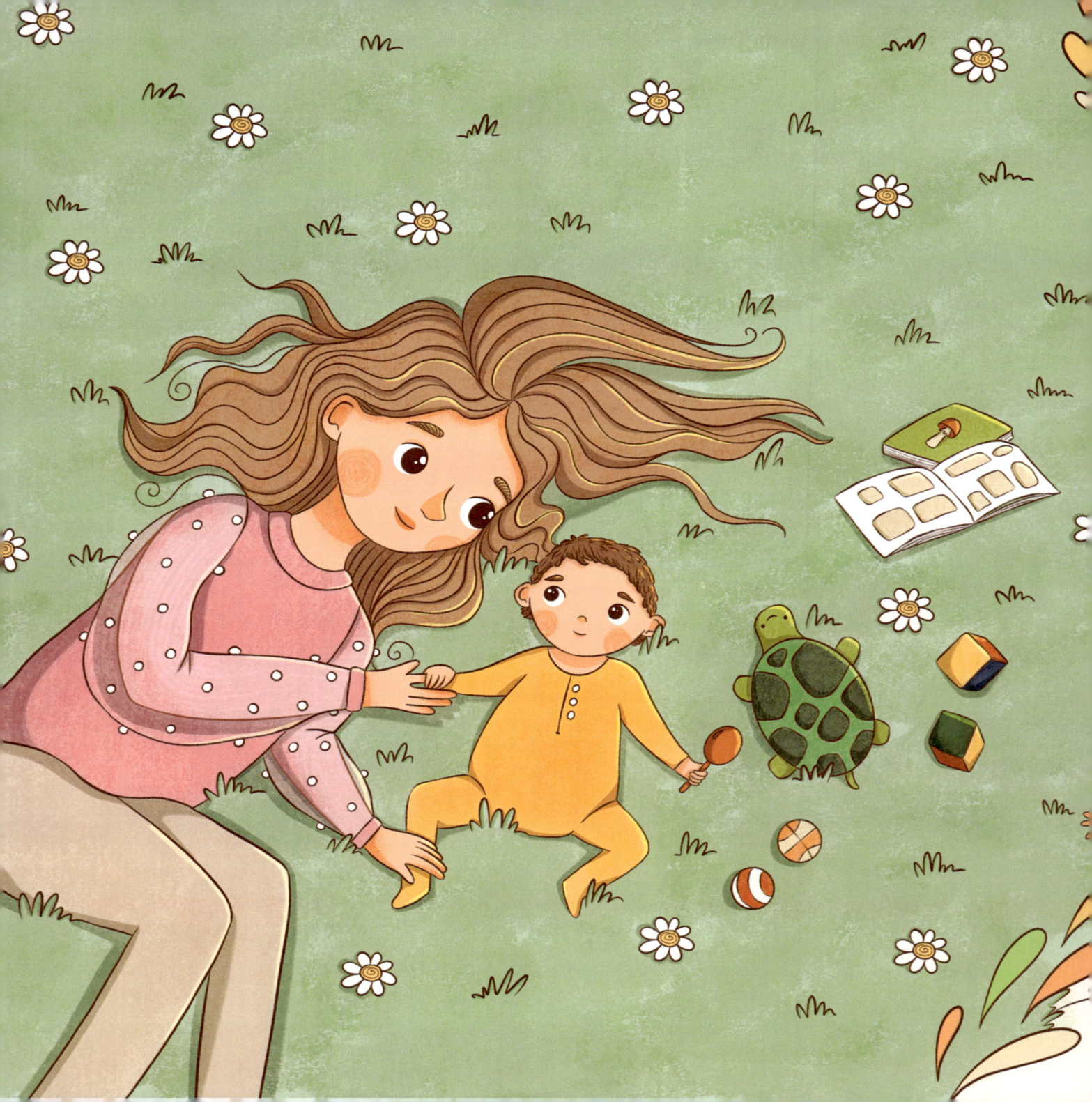

3-6 months:
Turn-taking
Vocalizations

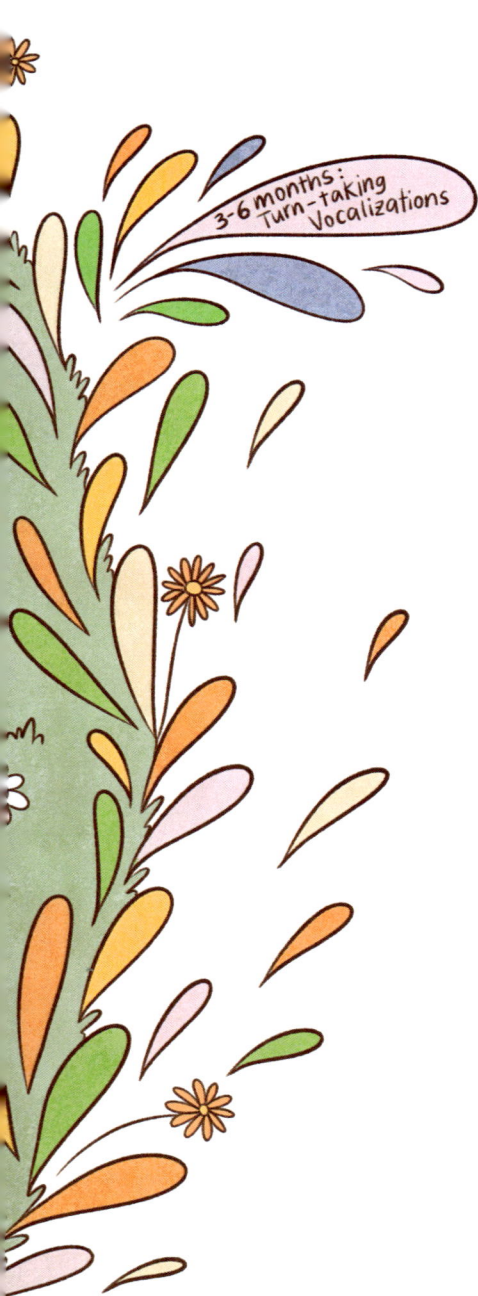

When I'm not napping,
I like to play peekaboo.
If you make a sound,
I'll repeat it to you.

Contact baby's pediatrician
and reach out to a
speech-language pathologist
at **6 months** if baby is not:

turning head towards sounds; looking at someone speaking
to them; smiling socially; cooing or making vowel sounds.

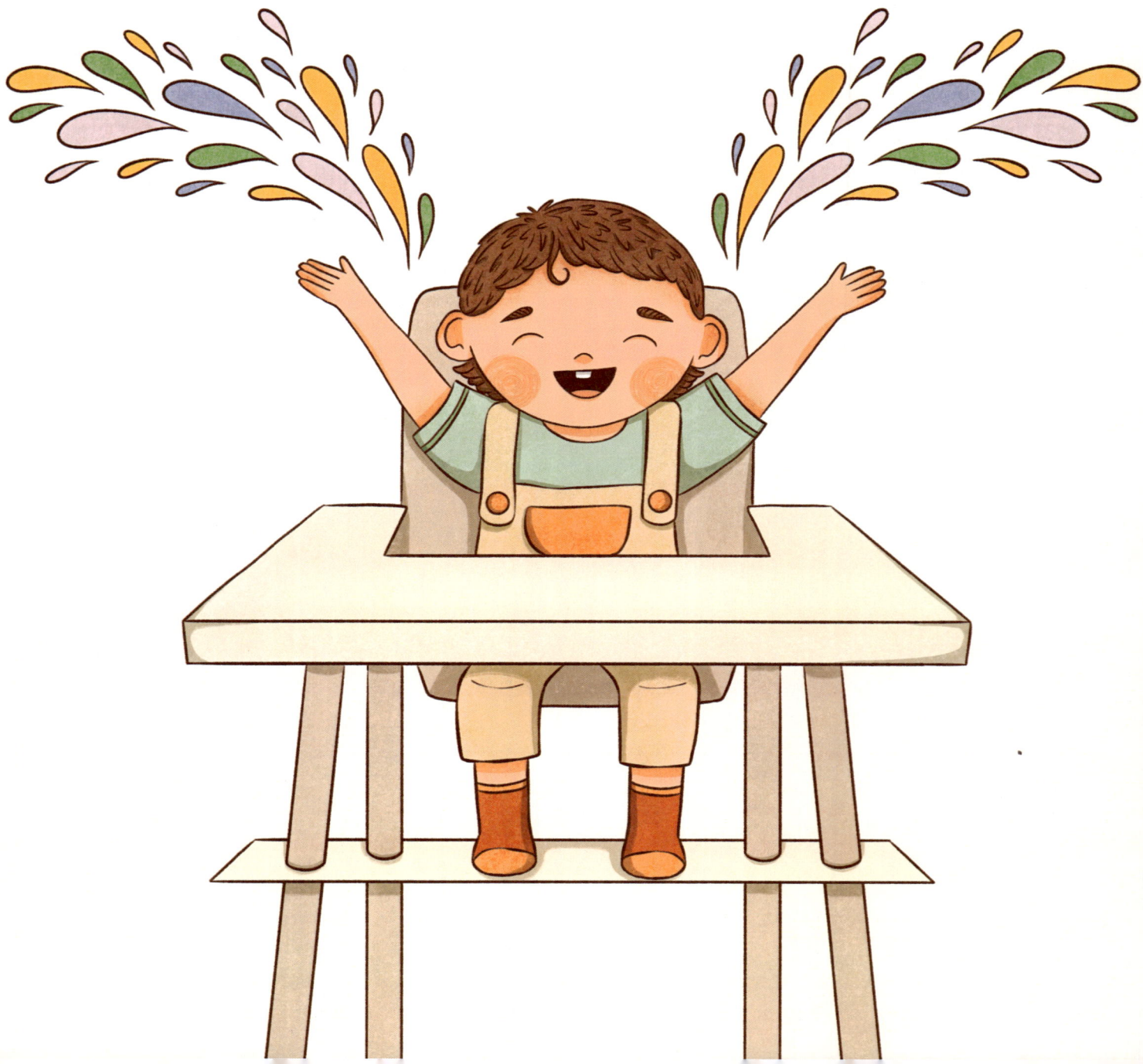

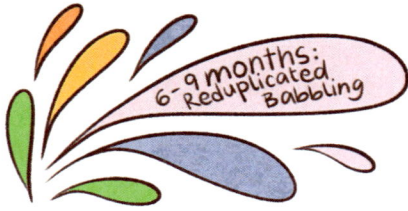

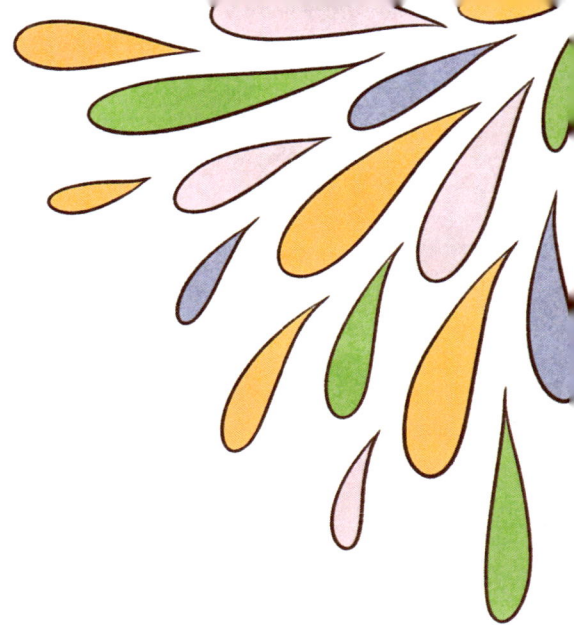

Mama and Dada,
Did you call my name?
Try it again;
I'm so good at this game!

Contact baby's pediatrician and reach out to a speech-language pathologist at **9 months** if baby is not: making eye contact; showing enjoyment with caregiver; responding to name; making consonant sounds.

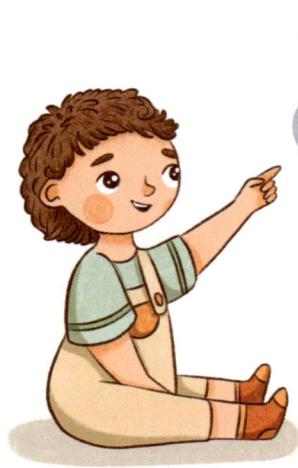

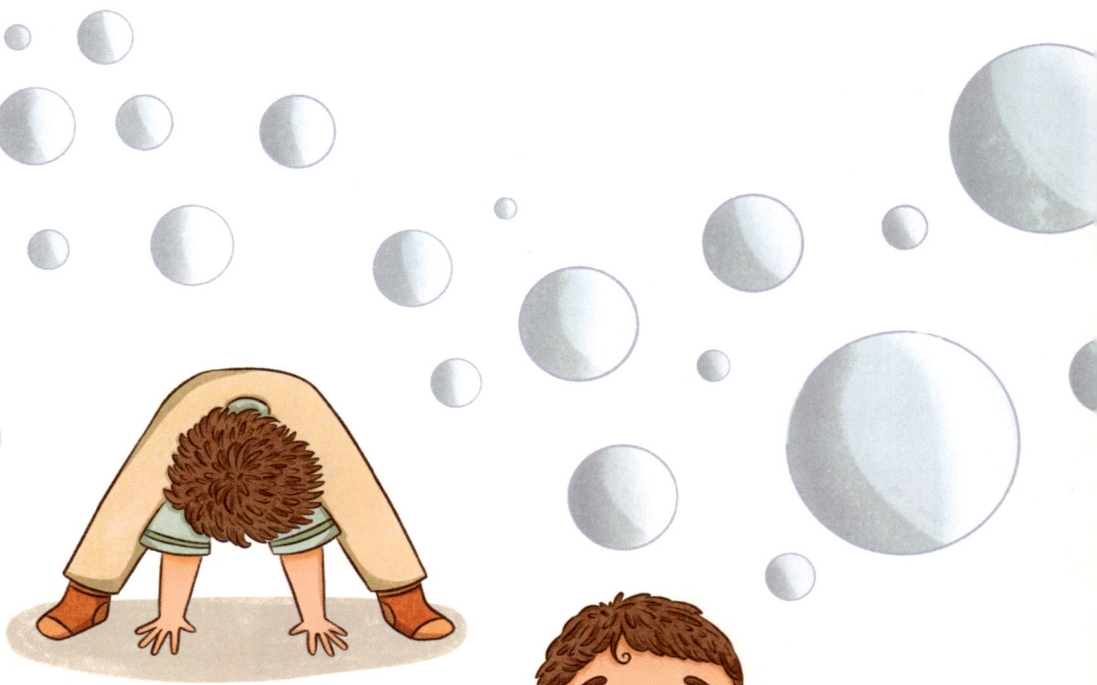

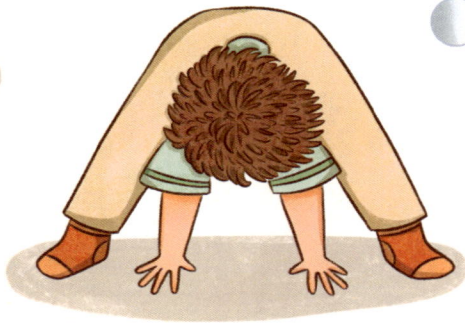

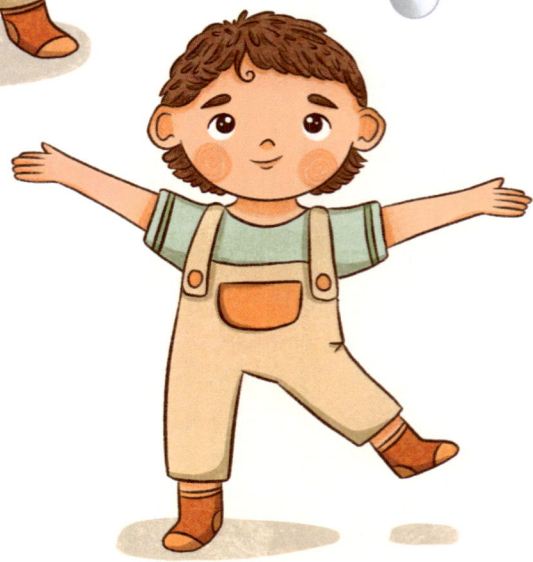

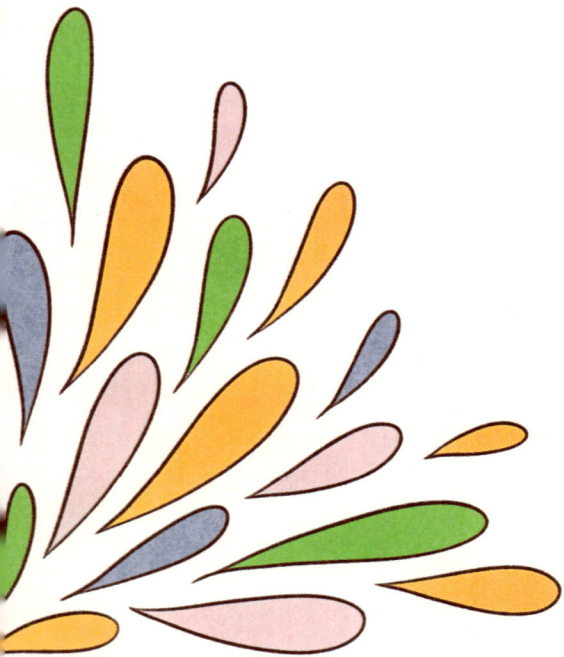

9-12 months:
Variegated Babbling

Look! I see bubbles!
I pop and I tap.
I beg you for more
as I giggle and clap.

Contact baby's pediatrician and reach out to a speech-language pathologist at **12 months** if baby is not: responding to name; babbling; using any gestures (e.g., reaching, waving, pointing, clapping).

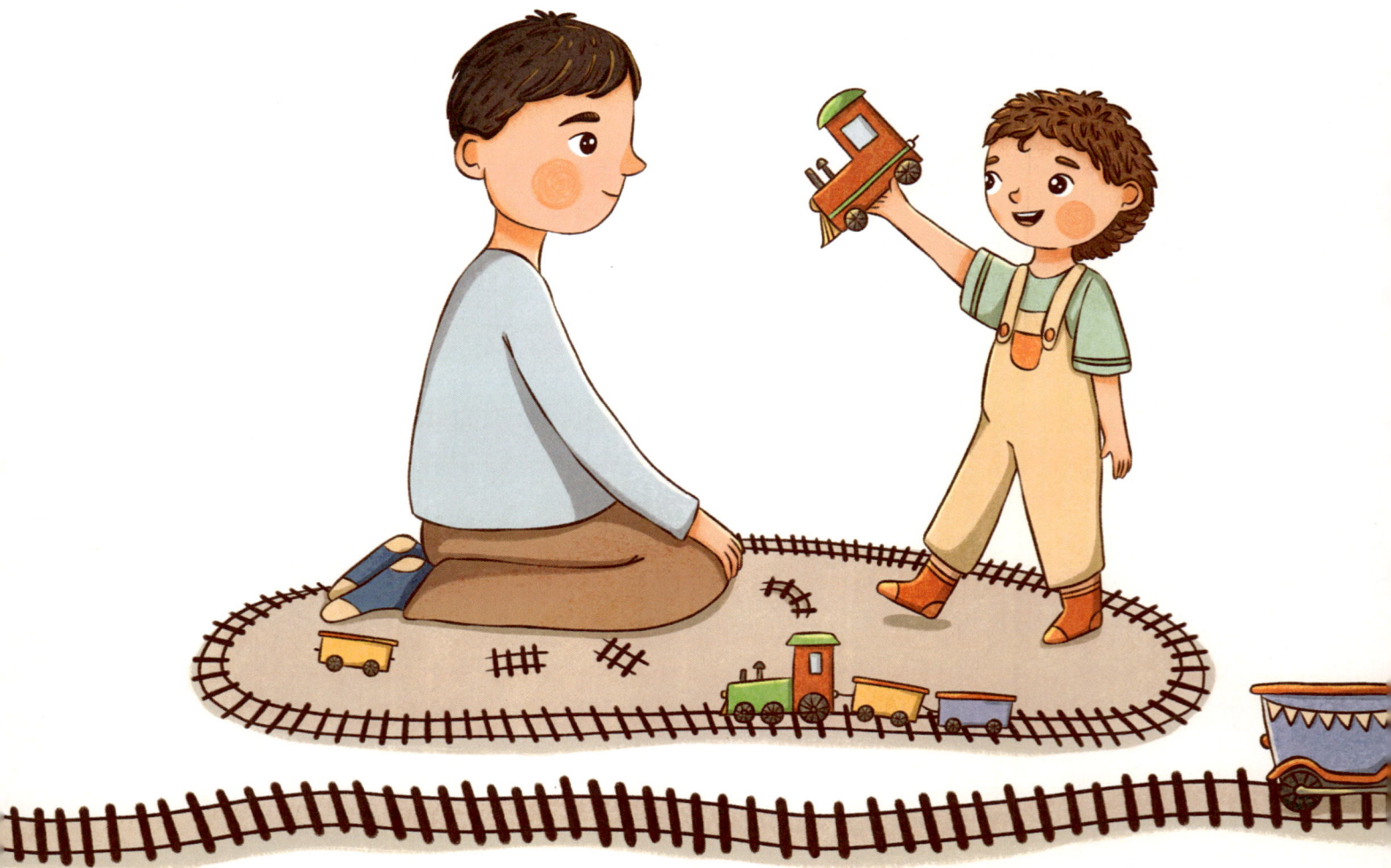

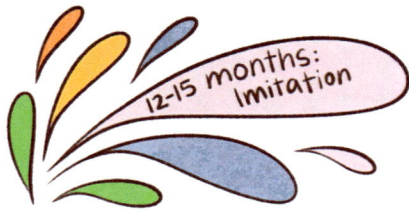

Mama's my best friend.
I love Dada, too.
He brought me a train
and we sang out, "Choo-choo!"

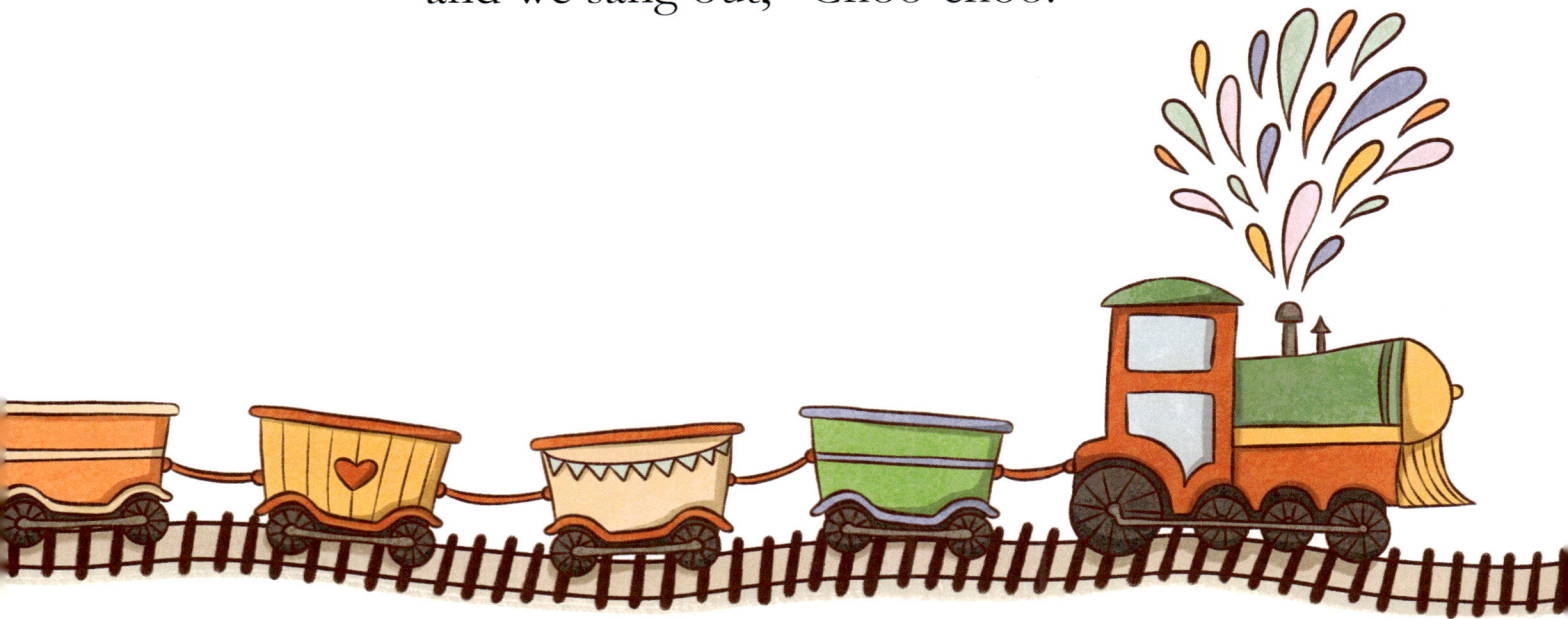

Contact baby's pediatrician and reach out to a speech-language pathologist at **15 months** if baby is not: showing understanding of common words and phrases (e.g., not following one-step directions); saying any words; using at least 3 consonant sounds (p, b, m, n, t, d, w, h).

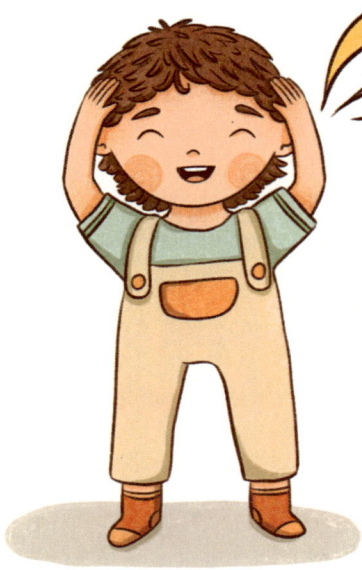

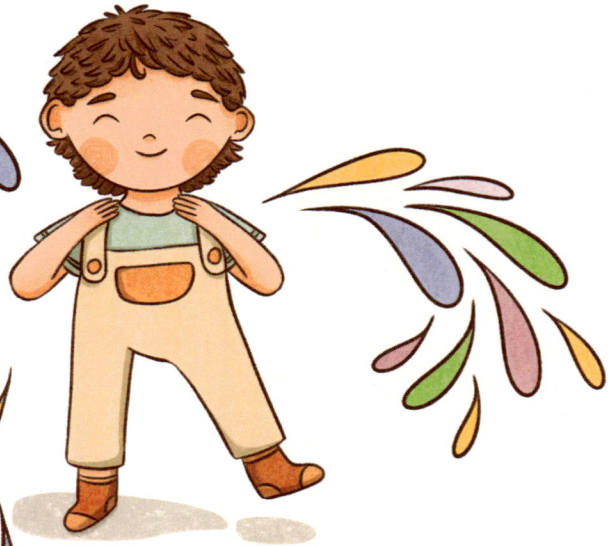

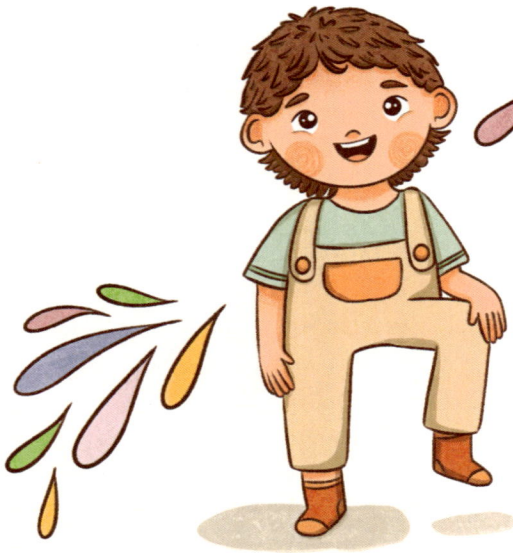

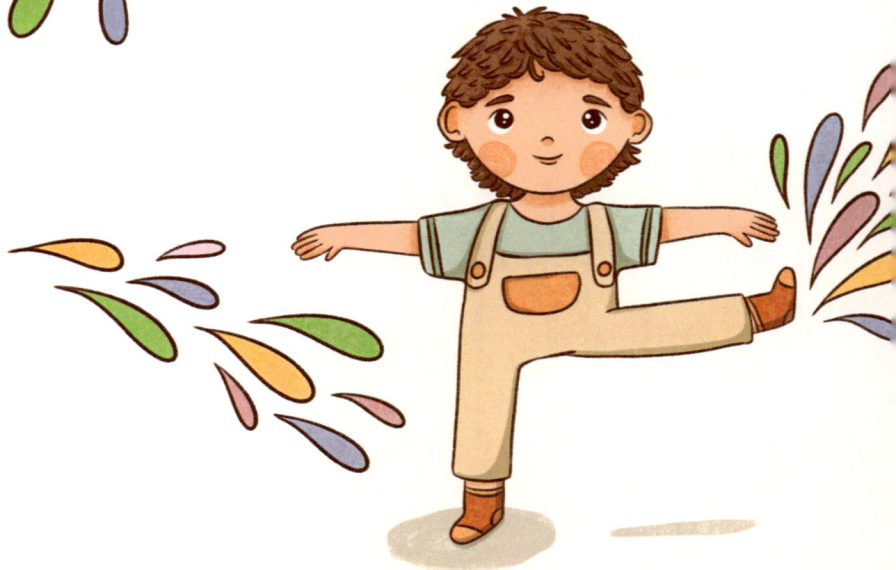

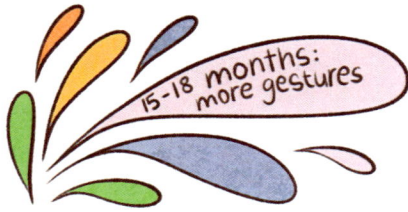

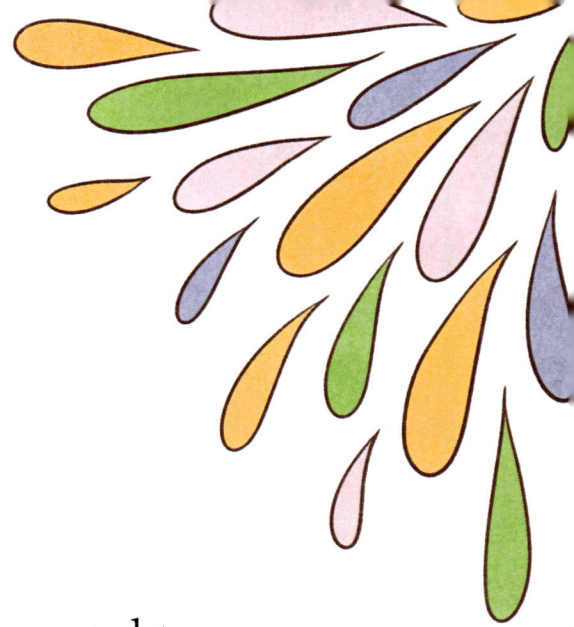

I reach for my head, shoulders, knees, and toes.
Sing to me, Mama, and I'll touch my nose!
Keep singing, Mama. I'll put on a show.
Until I get tired, and then I'll say, "No!"

Contact baby's pediatrician and reach out to a speech-language pathologist at **18 months** if baby is not: following simple directions; using at least 10 words; imitating simple actions and sounds.

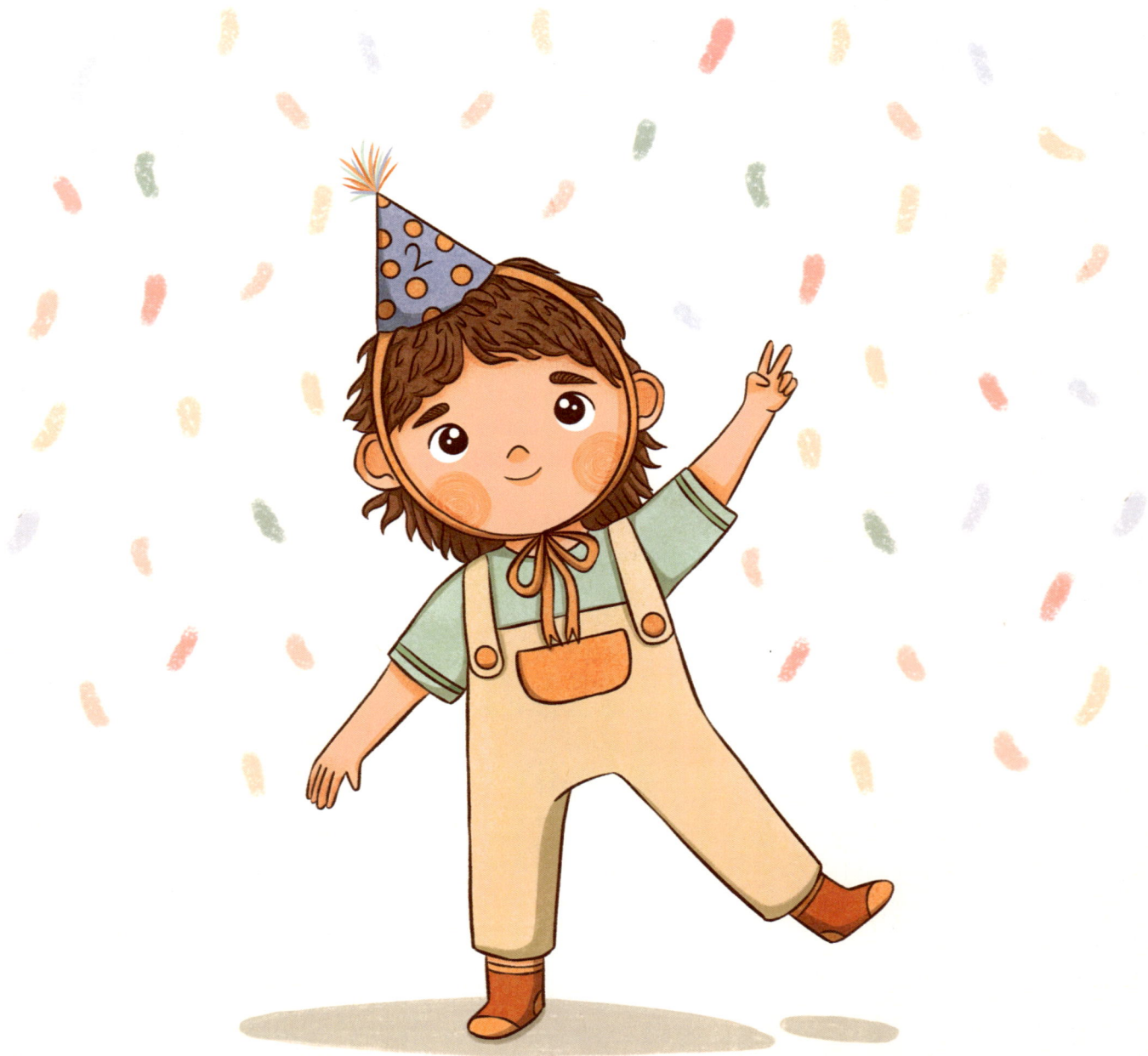

18-24 months: more words, less gestures

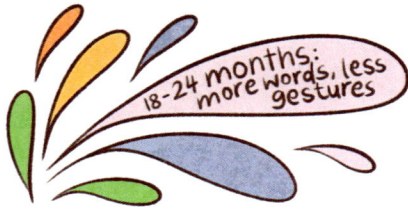

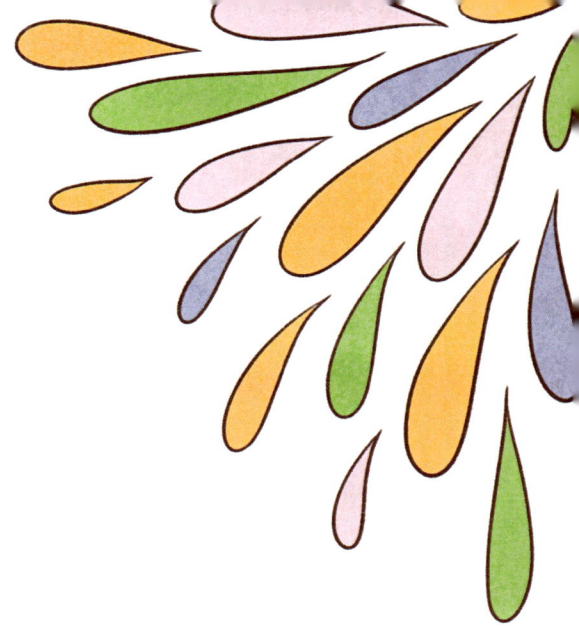

Mama, I'm growing.
Now I'm almost two.
I can answer your questions
to "Yes?" "No?" and "Who?"

Contact baby's pediatrician and reach out to a speech-language pathologist at **24 months** if baby is not: following one-step directions (e.g., get your shoes); using at least 50 words; using at least 5 consonant sounds (p, b, m, n, t, d, w, h).

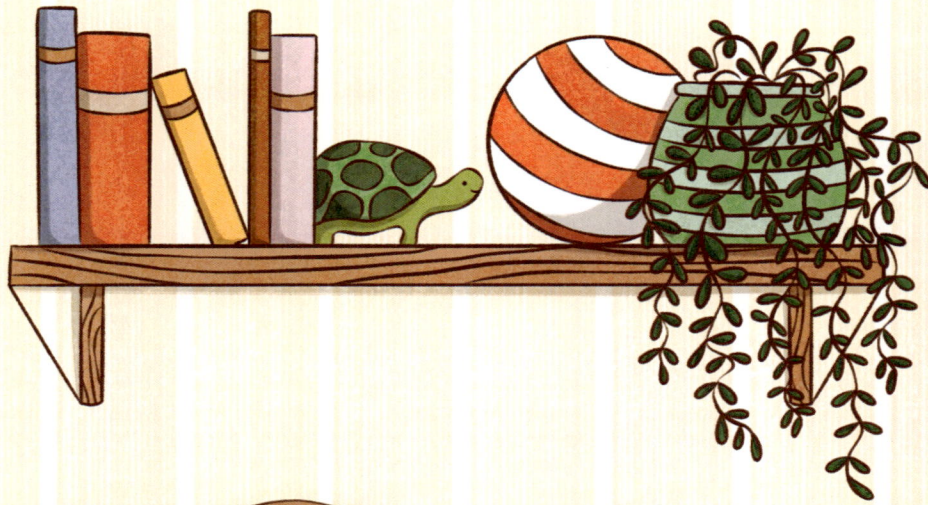

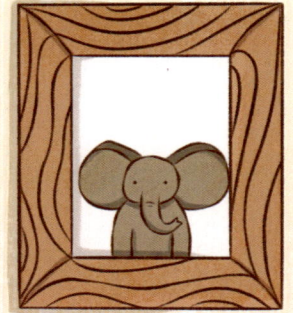

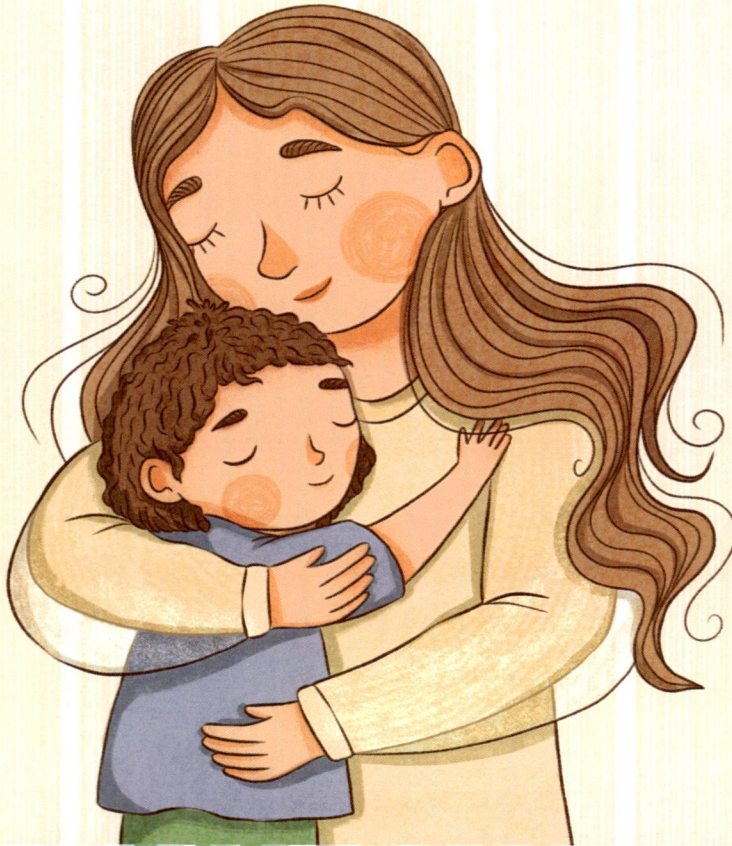

24-36 months: Robust Expressive Vocabulary

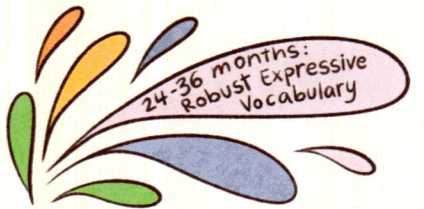

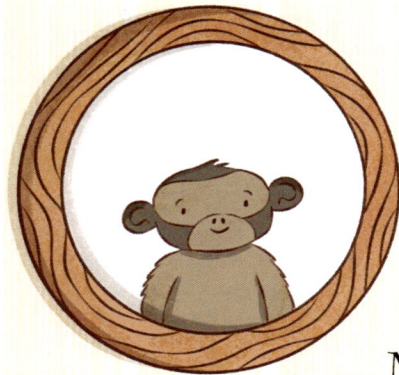

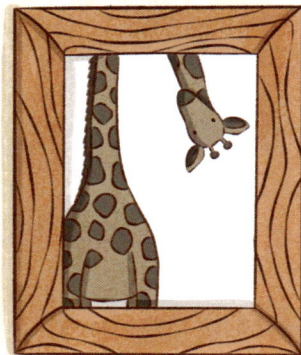

More time goes by,
and soon I will be three!
My favorite thing to say is,
"I love you, Mommy!"

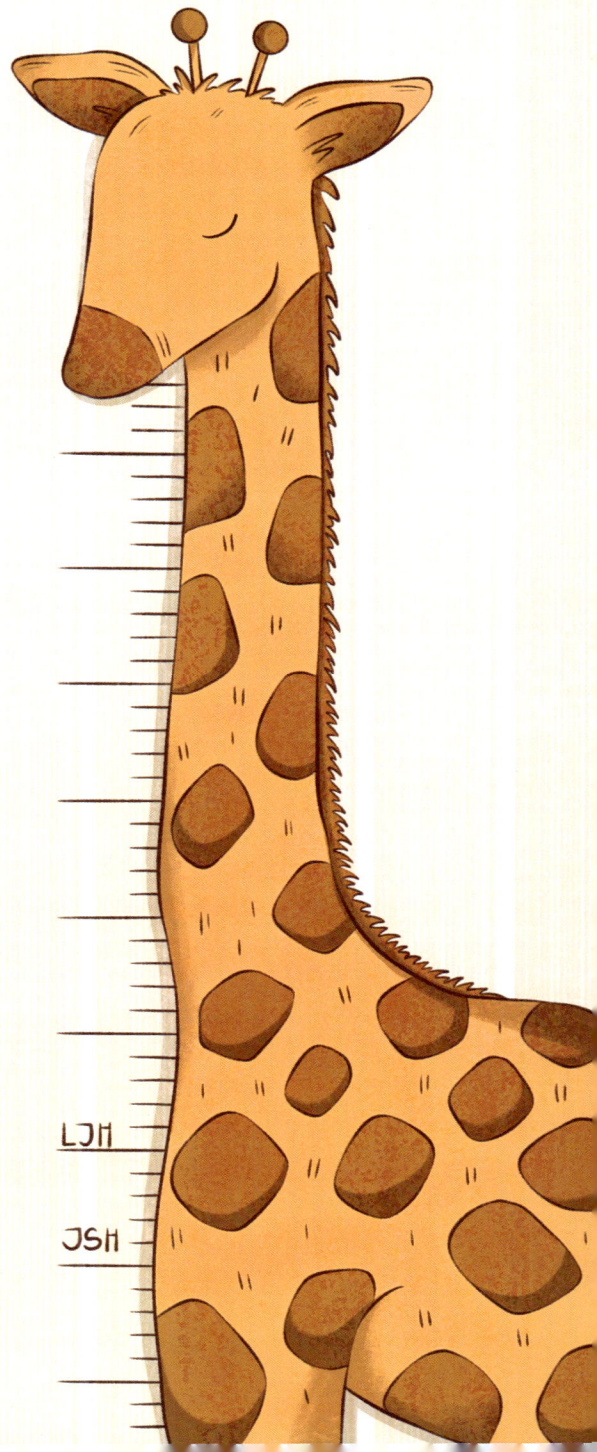

Contact baby's pediatrician and reach out to a speech-language pathologist at **36 months** if baby is not: following directions with simple concepts; using more words than gestures to communicate; or if baby is still in babbling stage, not combing words, and speech is less than 50% intelligible.

LJH

JSH

SPEECH AND LANGUAGE DEVELOPMENT

Birth – 3 months	- Recognizes familiar voice (e.g., mom and dad) since 27 weeks in womb - Startles to loud voice/sound - Turns head to voice/sound - Calms down when caregiver talks to them - Responds/vocalizes when talked to - Social smile - Vowel sounds and coos - Has different types of crying to signal different needs (sound reflexes)
3 – 6 months	- Enjoys social games and playful interactions with the caregiver (e.g., peekaboo, tickling, lap bounces) - Makes eye contact with people talking to them - Giggles/laughs - Expresses emotions (e.g., anger) with sounds other than crying (e.g., yelling, squealing, and shrieking) - Takes turn vocalizing - Consonant-vowel syllables shapes with /p, b, m/ sounds (e.g., puh, bah, muh)
6 – 9 months	- Responds to name - Joint attention emerges (e.g., attends to music) - Understands a few words and phrases (e.g., come here, stops momentarily to "no") - Communicates with vocalizations and eye contact - Reduplicated babbling (e.g., mamamama) - Emergence of baby sign language (e.g., milk, more) - Imitates some simple actions and sounds - May use some early gestures (e.g., gestures for 'up', reaching for items, pushing things away).
9 – 12 months	- Follows one step directions when prompted with gesture - Early gestures (e.g., pointing, waving, clapping) - Stops activity when told "no" - Bounces/vocalizes to music - Demonstrates variegated babbling (babbles a variety of consonant and vowels sounds) - Understands ~50 words and phrases - Imitates simple actions with nursery songs - Says one word by 12 months

American Speech and Hearing Association. Developmental Norms for Speech and Language.(2019).
Centers for Disease Control and Prevention. Learn the Signs. (2018).
Lanza and Flahive. Linguisystems Guide to Communication Milestones. (2008).

SPEECH AND LANGUAGE DEVELOPMENT

12 – 15 months	- Follows one step directions without gesture - Looks appropriately when asked questions such as,, "Where is the ball?" - Can say between 1-10 words - Produces immature jargon: babbling without real words with adult intonation - Uses 10 or more gestures (e.g., waves, points, claps, reaches to be picked up, smacks lips) - Imitates sounds in play (e.g., moo, vroom, aww, choo choo!)
15 – 18 months	- Points to identify common body parts and objects - Points to familiar people when named - Can say between 10-50 words - Speech is ~25% intelligible - Produces mature jargon: babbling with some real words - Imitates simple words (e.g., ball, mama, dada, up, boo!) - Emergence of saying "no."
18 – 24 months	- Makes choices when given two or more options - Follows simple two step directions - Uses words more often than gestures to communicate - Combines two words together (e.g., all done, mama help) - Can say between 50-300 words - Speech is 25-50% intelligible - Answers simple questions (yes/no?)
24 – 36 months	- Understands increasingly complex directions that include spatial concepts (e.g., on, off, under, big, little) - Follows 2-3 step directions - Gives first and last name - Can say between 300-1000 words - Produces phrases/sentences 2-3+ words - Displays advanced expressive vocabulary of nouns, verbs, descriptive words, and words for simple concepts (e.g., in, out, up, down) - Uses pronouns (e.g., I, me, you) - Echolalia and jargoning gone - Speech is 50-80% intelligible - Asks/answers simple questions (e.g., Who, What, Where, & What Doing?)

FETAL HEARING DEVELOPMENT

4 – 5 weeks embryo	Cells in embryo start to arrange themselves into baby's face, brain, nose, ears, and eyes.
9 weeks old embryo	Indentations appear where baby's ears will grow.
18 weeks old fetus	Baby starts to hear sound.
24 weeks old fetus	Baby is more sensitive to sound.
25 – 26 weeks old fetus	Baby responds to noises/voices in the womb.
27 weeks old fetus	Baby recognizes the sound of parent's voice, and prefers native language.

Healthline. Fetal Hearing Development: A Timeline. (2018).
Lozier Institute. Hearing in the Womb. (2023).

Dear Parents,

Every child's developmental journey looks a little different. But, if you're concerned that your child isn't meeting his/her milestones in an appropriate time frame, consult with your doctor and reach out to a speech-language pathologist. It is never too early.

You are doing great.

– Brenda L. Hwang

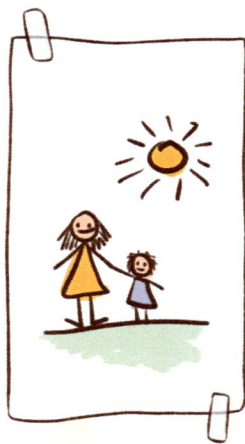

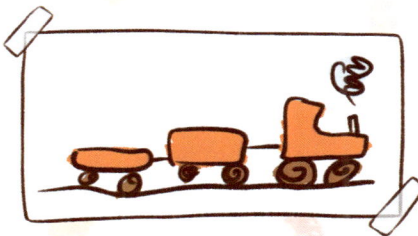

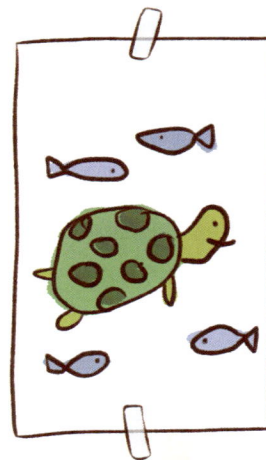

About the Author

Brenda Hwang is a speech-language pathologist, lactation counselor, and infant feeding specialist. During her post graduate training, she completed her fellowship specializing in early language intervention. Brenda is currently a doctoral candidate and plans to continue pursuing an advanced degree in serving the early intervention population in the areas of speech, language, and infant feeding disorders that pertain to lactation and breastfeeding.

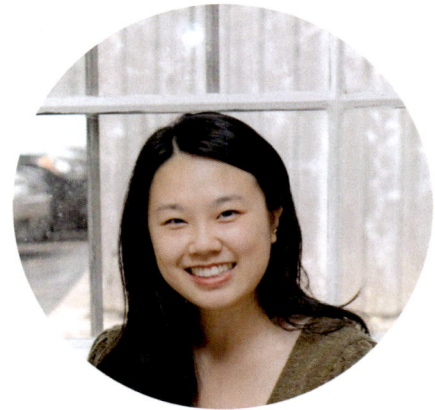

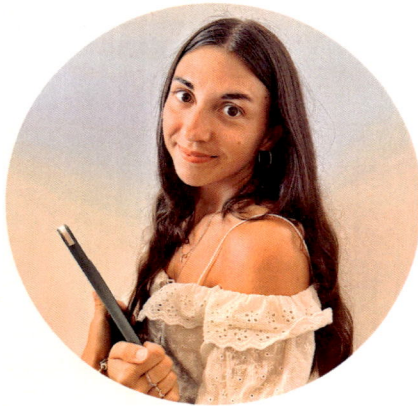

About the illustrator

Winona Kieslich (@winonaki) is a children's book illustrator from Germany. She started her journey in the world of digital illustrations while traveling around Australia. Drawing and being creative have always been very important for her. The art she creates focuses on whimsical and playful children's illustrations with a touch of magic.

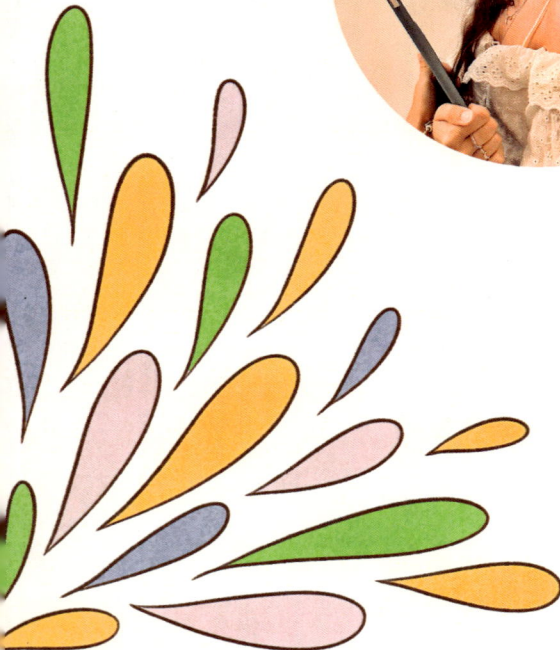

www.ingramcontent.com/pod-product-compliance
Lightning Source LLC
Chambersburg PA
CBRC091537260326
41914CB00022B/1647